Face

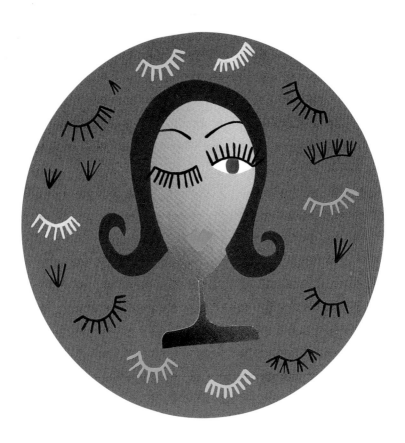

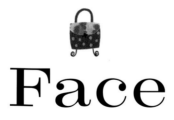

Face

100 makeup moves

Carol Morley & Liz Wilde

TIME
LIFE
BOOKS

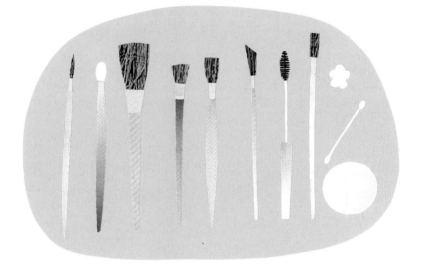

introduction

   Make maximum impact with minimum effort—it's easy when
you know how. Packed with 100 professional tips for a perfect face,
this little book tells you how to make the most of what you've got
and includes the secrets of everyday skin care and tips for those
times when you need a little extra help. Makeup advice covers clever
concealing, a better base, staying power, the perfect pout, and quick
fixes for ugly days. Put it all together and you've got the complete
guide to making sure you always look your absolute best!

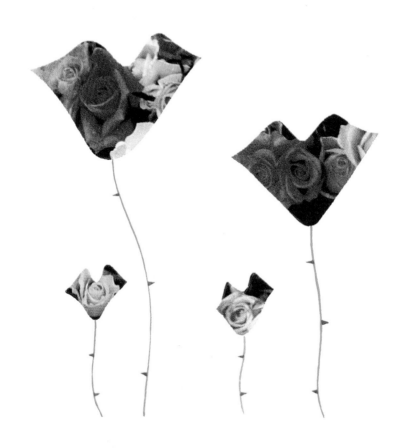

contents

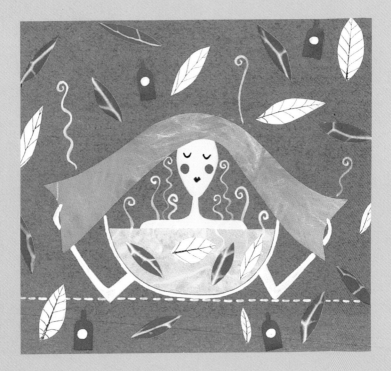

chapter 1

Skin savers

1 The most important thing you can do for your skin is to keep it clean. Before washing your face make sure your hands are clean so you don't transfer bacteria. Massage cleanser into your face, leave for a few seconds to dissolve impurities, then wipe away with a damp tissue or cotton ball. Follow with a splash of cool water to remove excess cream and rev up circulation, then pat dry with a soft towel.

2 Cleanse well before using a face mask or the skin-improving ingredients won't be able to reach your skin through the grime. Be generous—most masks should be spread on fairly thickly.

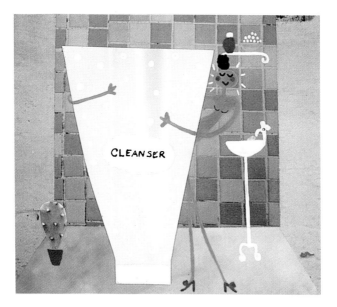

CLEANSER

3 **Don't know what skin type you have?** Look at your pore size through a magnifying mirror for the answer. If they're like craters you have oily skin; small pores mean dry skin; and a mixture of both indicates combination skin. Don't believe the hype about toners being able to close pores—it's one of those marketing myths used to make us part with our money. Some toners can temporarily tighten pores by dilating the capillaries, but the effect won't last beyond the front door.

4 **Pour mineral water into a spray bottle** and spritz your face after cleansing but before moisturizing. The water will plump up your skin and the cream will lock in the moisture for up to 12 hours.

5 **Using a toner after you've cleansed will refresh your skin.** Avoid alcohol-based toners even if your skin's oily—stripping your skin of grease will only encourage it to pump out more oil. Try using floral waters as toners. Available from drug stores, these are applied undiluted with a cotton ball. Choose witch hazel for oily and problem-prone skin, rose water for dry skin, and chamomile water for normal and sensitive skin. For a homemade toner, liquefy and strain a cucumber, pour into a spray container, and store in the refrigerator.

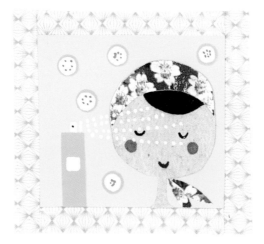

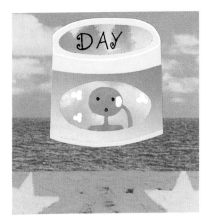

6 **Daytime moisturizing is about protecting your skin from the elements.** If your skin's dry, you need a rich cream to protect from moisture loss. If your skin's oily, a light, oil-free lotion will do the job without plugging your pores.

14

Nighttime moisturizing is about nourishing, so night creams are richer than day creams. Whatever the manufacturers would have you believe, it isn't essential that you match your day and night moisturizers—any brand that suits your skin will do.

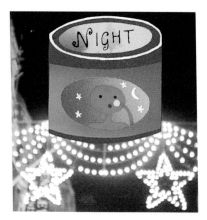

7 Facial scrubs help remove dead skin cells and surface grime, leaving skin feeling firm and smooth. Scratchy pads and brushes can be too abrasive, so choose a scrub with tiny granules that dissolve in water, and use once a week. Massage onto damp skin and rinse off. Make your own from any of the following:

- *Combine grapefruit juice and oatmeal into a paste.*
- *Add sugar to your cleanser and massage onto your skin.*
- *Mash together strawberries and oatmeal.*
- *Mix ground almonds with ground dried orange peel and a few drops of almond oil.*

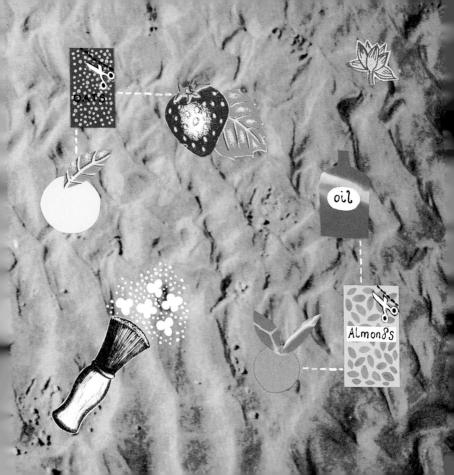

8 While you're asleep, a special skin growth hormone is released to boost collagen and keratin production (the proteins that make up your skin), and encourage cell turnover. Lose sleep and you're asking for dull, dry skin and deep, dark eyes. Try to squeeze in some extra shut-eye and you can help fight skin problems. It's not called beauty sleep for nothing.

9 Start the day with a quick detox drink. A glass of cooled boiled water to which you've added the juice of half a lemon will help to flush out all the impurities that your body has managed to pick up overnight.

10 Exercise won't just whittle your waist. As the heart starts pumping, oxygen races around your body bringing with it nutrients to feed your skin cells. The result is more collagen production, which improves the texture of your skin, and increased blood flow, which unclogs pores and dislodges grime. At the very least you'll get a healthy glow.

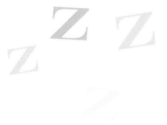

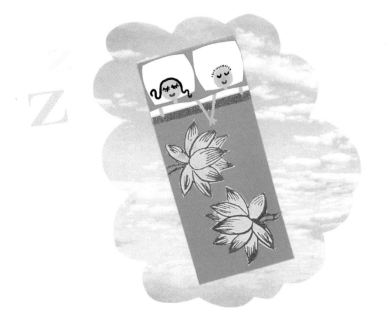

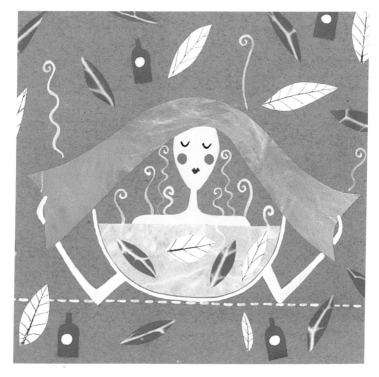

11 You get the same feel from steaming your skin as you do sitting in a sauna—deep-down clean from the bottom of every pore. Fill a bowl with near-boiling water and add a few drops of essential oil—choose lemon for oily skins, chamomile for dry, and mandarin for normal. Protect the thinner skin around your eyes by smoothing on moisturizer, then hold your face over the steam with a towel over your head. Follow with a face mask for the ultimate in dirt removal.

12 Drink about eight 8 oz glasses of water per day to help flush away toxins. Non-carbonated water at room temperature is best as it's most compatible with your body.

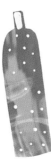
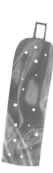
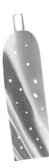
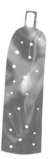

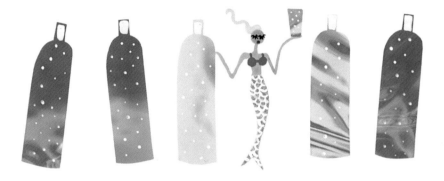

13 **Want to create a cheap facial?** Face masks are the easiest beauty treatment to make at home. All the following should be left on the skin for 10 to 15 minutes, then rinsed off with water.

- *Smooth on plain yogurt—it contains a form of lactic acid that works as a natural exfoliant.*
- *Mashed avocado pulp rubbed into the skin is a great moisturizing mask. Mayonnaise works well too (and can also be used on your hair for deep conditioning).*
- *A beaten egg white sprinkled with 1 teaspoon of vitamin C powder is a great skin saver.*
- *An egg white mixed with straw berries will absorb excess oil.*

14 Your body needs the right nutrients to make new skin. Base your diet on fresh foods like fruit and vegetables, brown rice and whole-wheat bread, grilled fish and chicken, and yogurt with live cultures.

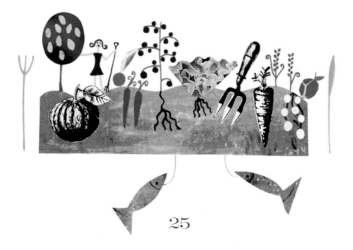

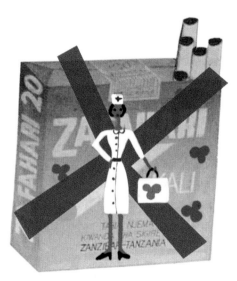

15 **Did you know that your skin renews itself every two to three weeks?** During your life you lose around 30 pounds of dead skin cells, which end up as household dust. More work for your duster, but the good news is any blemishes or slight scarring that you have won't last for ever.

16 **Gravity pulls your skin down, so when massaging in moisturizer work up and out toward your hairline.** Or copy the professional trick and lightly pat it on with your fingertips to increase circulation.

17 **Massage in your moisturizer and wait 10 minutes for it to sink in** before starting your makeup. Working on an oily face is the main reason for disappearing makeup and panda eyes.

18 **If you can't quit for your health, quit for your skin.** After the sun, smoking is the second major cause of premature wrinkles. Nicotine constricts the small blood vessels and decreases the flow of oxygen and nutrients to your skin. And all that sucking on cigarettes causes lines around your lips. Nasty.

19 Choosing a moisturiser used to be easy, but now you need a degree in science to understand all the jargon…

Antioxidants attack skin-aging free radicals present in atmospheric pollution. Vitamin A, C, and E neutralize free-radical damage from sun, pollution, and tobacco smoke.

Alpha and Beta Hydroxy Acids (AHAs and BHAs) work chemically to unglue old cells from the skin's surface and help new ones emerge, resulting in smoother, clearer skin.

Retinol is the purest form of vitamin A. It works deep within your skin where wrinkles form. Products containing retinol need to be used for eight weeks before you see results. It's worth the wait since sun damage such as discoloration will fade, and fine lines will smooth out.

Liposomes (also called Microspheres and Nanospheres) are tiny capsules containing the skin food found in cell membranes. They penetrate the skin and give nourishment exactly where it's needed.

Oxygen is the main source of energy for cell renewal. The skin's natural level drops with time, tiredness, and stress, resulting in a dull complexion. Pure oxygen molecules in moisturizing lotion are delivered directly to the skin.

20 Your skin is under attack from the environment 365 days a year. The sun burns, the cold chaps, pollution asphyxiates and prevents oxygen flow, and free radicals chip away at the skin's structure. Take cover with a moisturizer containing SPF15 and added antioxidants to protect against dermal damage.

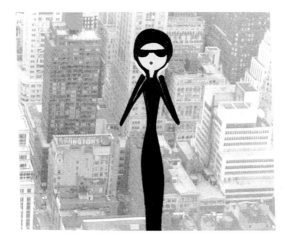

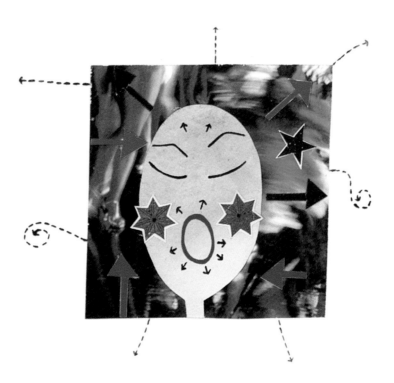

chapter 2

Special care

21 Cold weather can irritate even the hardiest skin. Swap your soap for a gentle cleanser, and moisturize more often to protect your skin from extreme temperatures. But beware of water-based moisturizers that can freeze on your face—oil-based creams freeze at a lower temperature and are much better for cold-weather protection.

22 Skiing holidays have never been more popular, but did you know about the danger of UVB rays reflecting off brilliant white snow? While sand reflects only 17 percent of these rays onto the body, freshly fallen snow returns a skin-baking 89 percent. Pack some serious protection to avoid sore faces (nothing under SPF25) and you'll also escape the dreaded goggle tan.

23 Extra-dry skin will love an intensive vitamin E boost. Splurge on a special cream or break open a vitamin E capsule (available from drugstores and most supermarkets) and smear it all over your face. This skin-friendly vitamin has lots of uses, including soothing chapped lips and moisturizing dry cuticles. Taken in pill form, vitamin E also increases your body's own natural sun-protection factor and strengthens the skin by fighting free radicals.

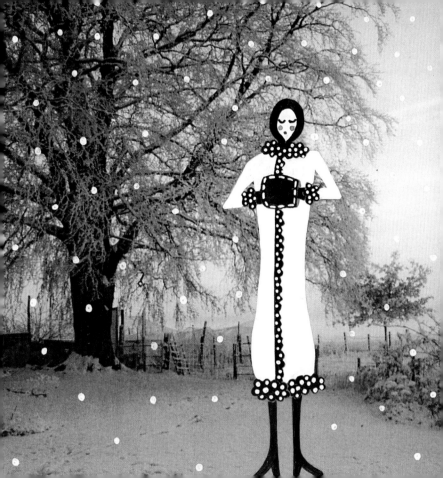

24 **Sun Safety:**

- *Always wear a high-protection sunscreen (no less than SPF15).*
- *Don't skimp on sunscreen; applied too thin it can lose up to half its protection.*
- *Reapply regularly, especially after swimming (even if it's waterproof).*
- *Rub in too hard and it won't work as well.*
- *Apply at least 30 minutes before going outside.*
- *Wear a hat and stay out of the hottest midday sun.*

25 **Before you venture into the sun, remember that the incidence of skin cancer is on the rise.** And some types can be fatal, including malignant melanoma, which is most common in young women. Why? It's thought the traditional beach vacation is the major culprit, and one bad burn might be all you need. Experts also agree that sun exposure is responsible for at least 80 percent of aging, and much of this harm is done before you're 18. UV light causes the usually straight and smooth collagen fibers in your skin to twist up. The result is skin that starts to sag, line, and wrinkle—especially facial skin, which is thinner than that on the rest of your body. So what do you do when no tan is a good tan, but most of us like a little color? The answer is fake it, don't bake it.

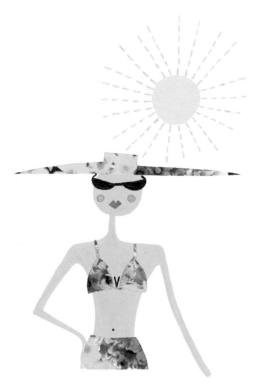

35

26 **Fly makeup-free to let your skin breathe,** and smooth on a rich moisturizer to protect against dehydration. A small spray bottle of water is in every model's carry-on for mid-flight moisturizing, as is a refreshing eye gel to de-bag tired eyes on arrival. Drinking plenty of water (avoid alcohol as this dehydrates you even more) and getting some shut-eye will make sure you breeze through arrivals fresh-faced. And if sleep proves elusive, invest in the model's other must-have—a large pair of sunglasses.

27 **If you're surrounded by technology every day** (as most of us are), an electronic ionizer is a worthwhile investment. It works by pumping out negative ions to counteract all the nasty stuff in the air. Just take a look at the amount of dust and dirt that an ionizer attracts.

28 **Central heating, especially forced hot air, can be very drying,** so save your skin by lowering the thermostat. Investing in a humidifier or keeping bowls of water or damp towels near your radiators will help to replace the lost moisture.

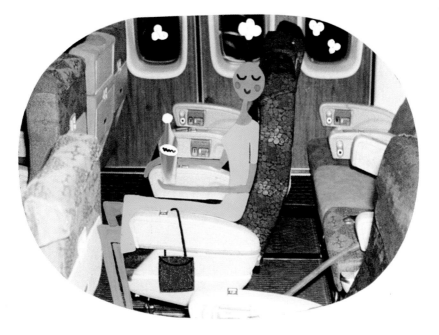

29 **Having trouble with your man's stubble?** Then show him how to shave properly. The closest shave is a wet shave using a swivel-headed razor and shaving cream. Lather with a brush that's been soaking in warm water, and massage into the face until all hairs are standing at attention. Always shave in the same direction as hair growth, and if this means every which way, then a sideways swipe is best. Finish off with a splash of cold water and a generous layer of moisturizer. Oh, and save any alcohol-based aftershave for later, after the skin has had a chance to calm down—otherwise he could end up with a nasty rash.

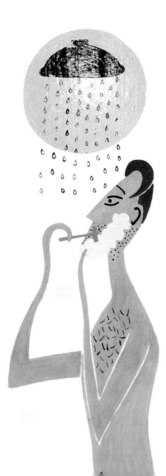

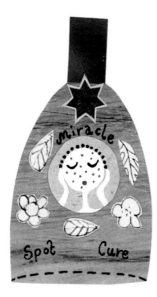

40

30 Bothered by a breakout?
There's no miracle cure for pimples, but regular dabs of antibacterial tea tree or lavender oil will help, as will a squeeze of toothpaste left on over night. Fight blemishes from the inside by getting enough sleep, eating healthily, and drinking lots of water. Eat garlic and onions (they might not win you friends but both are antibacterial) and high-fiber foods to kick-start sluggish circulation. Supplements thought to fight pimples are evening primrose oil, which helps balance hormones, and vitamin B, which slows down oil production (always follow the manufacturer's guidelines when using these supplements).

31 If your skin has more than the occasional eruption, it's worth seeking professional help to prevent future scarring. Your doctor has many potential cures that he or she can prescribe, and it's very rare for even the worst acne not to respond to the right treatment. Blemishes are usually fairly easy to cover with concealer, but for a professional quick fix, use eyedrops dabbed on with a cotton ball or swab. Makeup artists swear by this to calm things down in front of the camera.

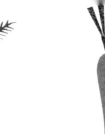

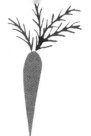

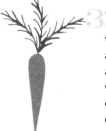

32 Raw vegetable juices contain vital vitamins, minerals, and enzymes, which can be absorbed into the bloodstream within 15 minutes. Blend and drink immediately so the juice doesn't oxidize and discolor.

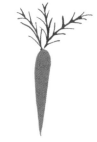

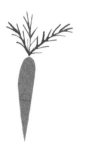

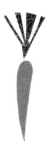

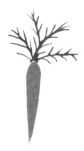

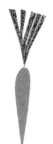

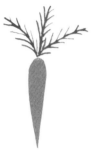

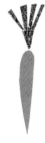

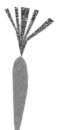

Carrot juice is at the top of your skin's wish list. Rich in vitamins A, B, C, D, and E, a glass will boost your immune system, fight infection, and protect against digestive disorders.

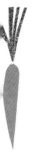

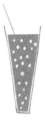

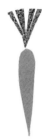

33 **Research tells us that 60 percent of us think our skin is sensitive,** but only 6 percent really have anything to moan about. But if you're one of the unlucky few, here's what to do.

• *The purer the product, the less likely your skin will be to react to it. If in doubt, switch to hypoallergenic and allergy-tested products.*

• *Patch-test products before using on your face by dotting a little on your neck and waiting 24 hours.*

• *Keep your skin care simple, avoid scrubs, masks, or moisturizers with fancy ingredients such as fruit acids, vitamins, or enzymes.*

• *Buy sunscreen products that are labeled "physical block." These con-tain titanium dioxide, which sits on the surface of your skin, rather than "chemical block," which sinks in and can irritate.*

• *If your skin flares up, splash with cool water and apply a soother like aqueous cream or aloe vera gel.*

34 **How to save your skin (and your head) the morning after a late night of partying:**

• *Going to bed in your makeup is not an option—it will clog up your pores. And failing to remove your mascara can cause your eyelashes to break. Special makeup removers are best, but in an emergency any moisturizer will do the job.*

• *Take a large dose of vitamin C with*

a 20 oz glass of water before you go to bed.

- Avoid caffeine and sip green tea instead. Stimulating and reviving, it has been known to clear many a hungover head.
- Sprinkle a few drops of essential oil into your bath (eucalyptus or rosemary works well) then lie back and relax.
- A hangover means you're dehydrated inside and out. Drink lots of mineral water and treat your skin to a moizturising face mask.

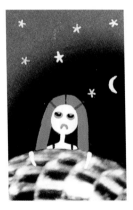

35 **If your skin needs a treat, try one of these homemade massage oils,** they penetrate more deeply into the dermis than creams—and the smell will soothe your brain too. Mix 5 teaspoons of any vegetable oil with no more than 15 drops of one essential oil. Choose the right one to suit your skin type.

Lavender possesses antiseptic properties and is beneficial for oily, blemished skins.

Geranium helps to balance combination skins.

Patchouli softens and helps to soothe dry skin.

36 **A regular face massage will bring blood to the surface of your skin to nourish cells and tone muscles.** You can't do anything to remove lines that are already there, but you can help to prevent new ones from developing. Choose a facial oil to suit your skin type and massage in for at least five minutes using small, light, circular movements with your fingertips.

37 **Exercise will do wonders for your complexion,** but don't do your aerobics in full makeup. Wash your face before your workout so your skin will be free to breathe and sweat will not block your pores.

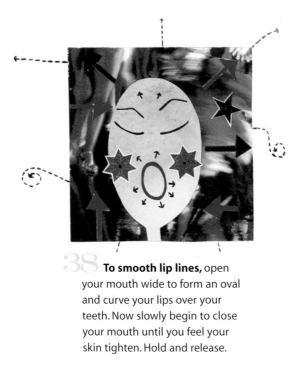

38 **To smooth lip lines,** open
your mouth wide to form an oval
and curve your lips over your
teeth. Now slowly begin to close
your mouth until you feel your
skin tighten. Hold and release.

39 **Give your face a twice-weekly workout to tighten up muscles and prevent signs of premature aging.**

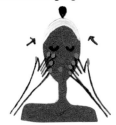

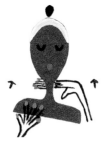

1. To smooth cheeks, using your first and second fingers, stroke up from chin to temple—being careful not to pull the skin. Repeat 20 times.

2. To sharpen up the jawline, lightly slap yourself under the chin with the back of one hand. Repeat 30 times.

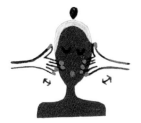

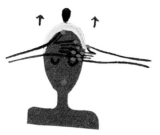

3. To firm the mouth and chin, start with gentle massage movements around the corners of your mouth, then alternating hands, stroke up from your chin to nostrils. Repeat 20 times.

4. To lift the area around the eyes, use your middle fingers and, starting on both sides of your nose, smooth up towards the bridge, out along your eyebrows, down your cheekbones, and back to your nose. Repeat 10 times.

40 **As far as skin damage is concerned, prevention is always better than cure,** but it's nice to know that there is a range of treatments out there that can help you to hold back the years.

Collagen injections plump out lines and wrinkles and lessen the appearance of frown lines. Either synthetic collagen or your body's own fat is used, but the results are temporary since the collagen is absorbed back into the body after about three months. Follow-up treatments are needed.

Skin peels remove the outer layers of wrinkled skin to reveal the softer, younger-looking skin beneath.

High concentrations of alpha hydroxy acids are applied to your skin; the results depend on the strength of the solution used.

Laser treatments remove the outer layers of damaged skin, including age spots and uneven skin tone. The results are good and far less painful than plastic surgery.

Nonsurgical face lifts tone the facial muscles using electronic equipment. A low frequency microcurrent is delivered directly to the skin, lifting the face and improving skin texture. A course of treatments will be needed and the results are temporary so you'll need to keep going back.

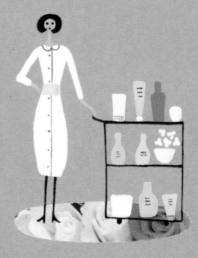

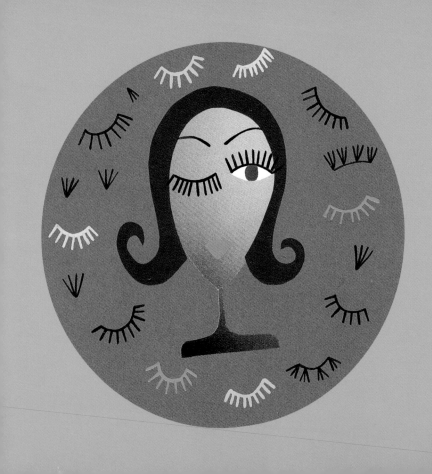

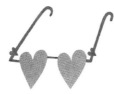

chapter 3

Bright eyes

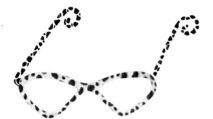

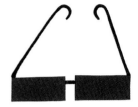

41 **Whether you're choosing expensive prescription glasses or cheap sunglasses,** here's how to find the most flattering frames.

• *Don't choose glasses that are the same shape as your face.*

Square faces should avoid angular frames, and round faces should steer clear of circular glasses.
• *Your eyebrows should line up with the top bar of your glasses.*
• *Your eyes should appear exactly in the middle of each lens or you'll end up looking cross-eyed.*

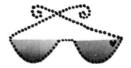

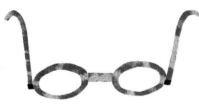

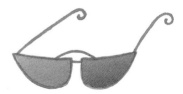

• *Make sure that the glasses you choose are comfortable and a good fit—that means they don't sit heavily on your cheeks or pinch the bridge of your nose and leave nasty marks on your face. If you're buying prescription glasses, the optician will be able to adjust the frames to suit the shape of your face so that you will get a perfect fit.*

42 **Sparkling eyes are a sign of a healthy diet** that includes vitamins A (carrots, red and yellow peppers, cantaloupe), B2 (milk and dairy foods, whole-grain bread), C (citrus fruit and juices), antioxidants (leafy deep-green vegetables) and zinc (meat, seafood, and whole grains). One of the signs of a vitamin A deficiency is dry eyes and difficulty seeing in dim light. A lack of vitamin B2 can cause eye irritation, and vitamin C strengthens the structure of capillaries in and around the eye. Research has shown that eating leafy green vegetables five times a week protects against blindness in old age, and zinc helps the eye use vitamin A to keep the retina healthy.

43 **Don't rely on whitening drops to brighten tired eyes.** Used too often, they can cause the capillaries to dilate permanently and can actually make your eyes look redder.

44 **Much kinder than chemicals, the herb eyebright is perfect for perking up your peepers.** Make your own infusion by mixing 4 tablespoons of the fresh plant or 2 tablespoons of dried herb with 2 cups of hot water. Allow it to cool, strain, pour into a bottle. Use to moisten cotton pads, then place them over your closed eyelids and relax for 10 minutes. Keep refrigerated and use within a week.

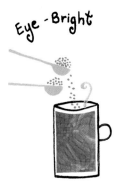

Eye - Bright

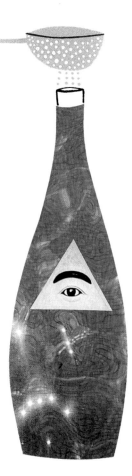

57

45 Just about anything cold will help to shrink baggy eyes. Try ice cubes wrapped in a plastic bag, or keep two stainless steel teaspoons in the refrigerator to place over your eyes. Other home-made de-baggers include cold slices of cucumber or raw potato and chilled camomile tea bags. And keep your eye cream or gel in the refrigerator for double-duty beauty.

46 The best concealers for under-eye shadows are light reflective, which means they bounce light off the problem. Apply concealer after foundation so you cover anything that's still visible, and gently pat along the darkest area before blending with your fingertip. Don't go lower than the bone under your eye, and add a dot at the inner corner for instantly brighter eyes. Save stick concealers for hiding more obvious blemishes as the sticks tend to dry into any fine lines. The result? Wrinkles before your time.

47 The skin around your eyes is the thinnest on your face and your usual moisturizer can block oil glands and cause puffiness. Invest in a lightweight eye cream and apply by gently tapping it inside the socket line and along the bone under your eye. Don't go any closer or it could get into your eyes and cause irritation.

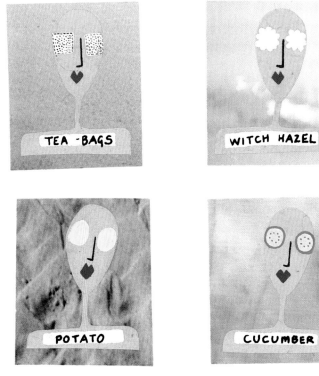

TEA - BAGS

WITCH HAZEL

POTATO

CUCUMBER

48 Well-shaped eyebrows are worth hours spent on makeup.

To do a good job you need sharp tweezers. (Revive blunt ones by running sandpaper over the inner edges.) If you have a low pain threshold, smooth a baby's teething gel over the area first to numb your skin. Pluck one hair at a time, concentrating underneath the brows, but if you've got odd stragglers above, there's no harm in yanking them out, too. But be warned—it's going to hurt. To groom, use clear mascara or spritz a little hair spray onto an eyebrow comb and then quickly brush through your brows.

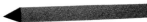

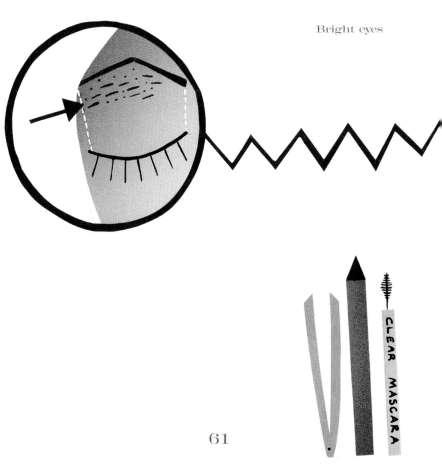

Bright eyes

61

49 **Two thin coats of mascara will look more natural than one thick one.** And adding a little extra just on the outside edges of the eyes will lengthen your lashes and open up your eyes. Light lashes always look better with brown mascara, and even dark lashes look softer in deep brown rather than basic black.

Long Lashes

50 **False eyelashes come in strips and clusters.** Keep it natural by just pressing on one small cluster of false lashes at the outside corners of your eyes. Squeeze a little glue onto the base and use tweezers for perfect placement. Then apply mascara to join you and your false lashes together; fill in any gaps with a little liquid eyeliner. For a fuller effect, strip lashes can be cut to the correct size. Apply glue along the base, then position the strip and fix the middle before gently pressing down both ends.

51 **Since the days of ancient Egypt,** eyeliner's been used to make eyes look bigger and lashes thicker.

Pencil blends easily for a subtle effect but fades quickly.

Powder eye shadow can be applied dry for soft definition. Dampen your brush and you'll get a stronger, longer-lasting line.

Liquid is tricky to master but is worth the effort—your line will last a lot longer than the others.

Pen eyeliner is an easy-to-use liquid that goes on like a felt-tip pen and dries to a smudgeproof color.

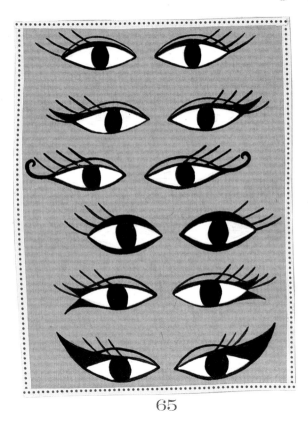

65

52 **Choosing an eye shadow is tricky business.** Don't try matching a shadow to your eye color—it's a contrasting, not similar, shade that will make your eyes stand out. Whatever color you choose, think in terms of three. A dark shade to line and define the crease, a medium shade on the lid, and a light one to highlight brow and inner eye. You also have to choose between cream or powder. Creams come in jars, wands, tubes, and pencils and give a wash of moist color. Use over foundation to avoid creasing. Powder comes in more color choices and is easier to use. A little face powder on your eyelids first will help it stick.

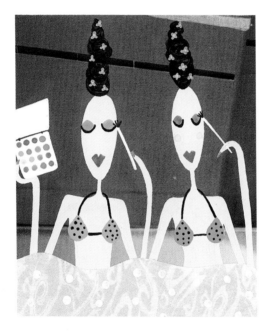

53 **Invest in a special oil-free eye-makeup remover** that won't irritate the delicate skin around your eyes. And always remove your contact lenses before taking off your eye makeup.

54 **The skin around your eyes is the first to wrinkle.** Fight back with a special eye cream designed to combat wrinkles, and apply morning and night. And always wear shades in the sunshine to prevent squinting.

55 **How often should you have your eyesight tested by an optometrist?** Experts say every two years, but you should go more often if you have any problems.

56 **Working at a computer for long periods can result in red eyes.** The static from your screen attracts dust from the atmosphere to the area right in front of your eyes. Invest in a special screen cover and a mini-ionizer to sit on your desk.

57 **Bloodshot eyes can happen for many reasons.** The main culprits are allergies, lack of sleep, or looking at a computer screen all day. If you suffer from sore, red eyes, try bathing them twice a day with a saline solution until they clear. You can make your own saline solution at home by dissolving $\frac{1}{2}$ a teaspoon of salt in 1 cup of mineral water.

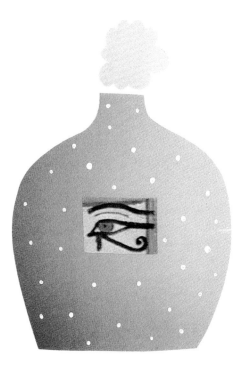

58 **Fed up with being asked if you've just had a good cry?**
Puffy eyes can mean waste retention (cut down on salty, spicy foods, caffeine, and alcohol), poor sinus drainage (sleep with an extra pillow) or toxin buildup (drink about 8 glasses of water a day to flush out your system). For an early-morning fix, soak two cotton balls in cold milk, place over your eyes and lie down for 10 minutes. Or if you are short of time, tap them away using your middle finger. Just one minute working lightly along the under-eye area moving from one corner to the other should be enough to calm even the puffiest of eyes down.

59 **Dark circles are caused by poor circulation, toxin buildup, lack of sleep—or bad luck.** If you constantly look like you haven't been to bed, the skin around your eyes is probably extra thin, which allows the underlying blood vessels and veins to show through. Cold compresses (cucumber and raw potato are the cheapest) will temporarily shrink blood vessels to lighten eyes. Invest in a concealer to brighten the area.

60 **Eyes too tired to carry on?**
Close them and cup the palms of your hands over each eye for at least one minute. A quick rest in the dark will do them worlds of good.

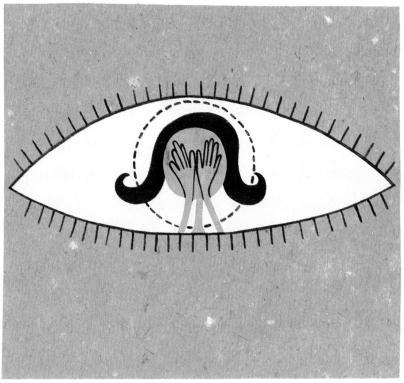

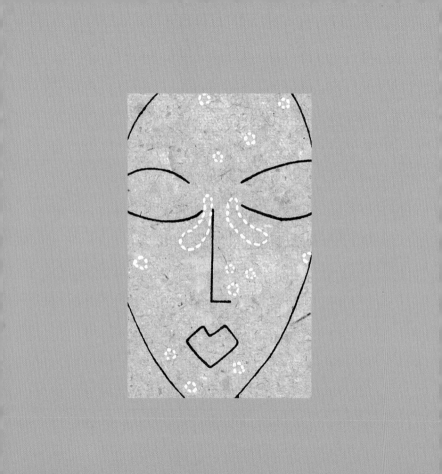

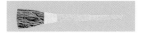

chapter 4

Makeup moves

61 Most people will see your makeup in daylight, so don't put it on in a dark corner of your (artificially lit) bathroom. The best place to put on your makeup is in front of a window, but for winter mornings, think about investing in a mirror with special bulbs that give off full-spectrum light.

62 Fed up spending time on your makeup only to have it disappear by lunchtime? The trick to achieving long-lasting makeup is to layer wet and dry textures. This means using powder over creamy concealer and foundation, and powder blusher over a cream one in a natural or matching shade. Before applying eye shadow, prime your eyelids with a little face powder pressed on with a puff to absorb oil. Using a lip pencil, fill in the whole lip area before brushing lipstick over the top; this will give it something to grab on to. Two fine coats of a water-resistant mascara will last longer than one clumpy coat. The main reasons for makeup not lasting are too much moisturizer, which will cause color to slide, and fiddling with your face.

63 The quickest way to light up your face when there's no time for messing around with makeup? Dress in light-colored clothing. It will reflect light up and onto your skin.

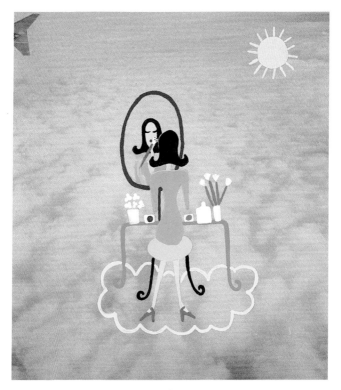

64 Using the right tools for the job is as important as using the right makeup. The ones you get free with most cosmetics are tricky to use and won't give good results. Invest in the five essential brushes: a concealer brush, eye-shadow brush, eyeliner brush, blusher brush, and lip brush. Buy them where you buy makeup, or try an art supply store for a wider selection of brushes. Make sure they feel soft and that the bristles aren't loose. Keep makeup brush-es clean by washing in a mild detergent whenever they get a build-up of color. Rinse well. Squeeze out excess water, reshape the bristles, and let dry overnight on a towel.

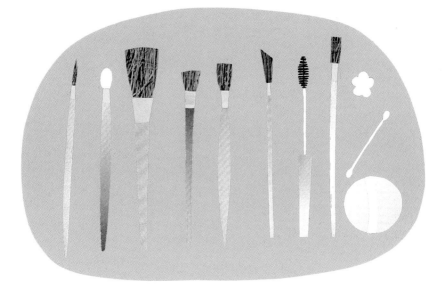

65 **The right shade of foundation should fade into your skin.** The best way to choose a base is to dot three different colors onto your face just above your jaw. The one that disappears is the one that you should buy.

66 **Got carried away applying your makeup?** Lighten up too heavy foundation or powder by spraying your face with a fine mist of water and then blotting with a tissue. Concealer that's caked will loosen up with a tiny dab of moisturizer, and too much eye shadow or blusher will look a whole lot less with a sweep of loose, translucent powder over the top.

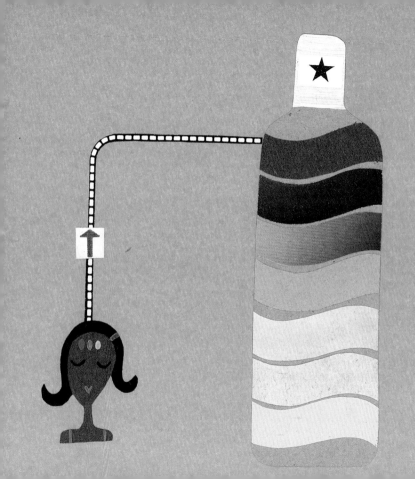

67 **Concealer is basically extra thick foundation** that comes in jars, sticks, and tubes. For the best all-around hiding, choose a stick concealer that gives good coverage and stays put once it's powdered (although this may be too heavy for the delicate under-eye area). The most common concealer mistake is using a shade that is too light, which only accentuates what you're trying to hide. Go for a yellow-based one that's only one or two shades lighter than your natural skin tone. Applying concealer with a small, firm brush will ensure perfect application. Paint over blemishes, birthmarks, and broken capillaries; blend edges; and then set by pressing on a yellow-toned powder with a velour puff. Use a large brush to dust away any excess and you can be sure your imperfections will stay hidden away all day.

68 **Natural makeup doesn't have to mean shades of beige.** Today's textures mean even bright colors come in wearable transparent formulas that give a sheer wash of color. The secret of wearing color on your eyes is to choose just one.

69 **Groom unruly eyebrows with a touch of clear mascara,** or squirt a little hairspray on to an eyebrow comb and brush them up. They'll stay in place all day.

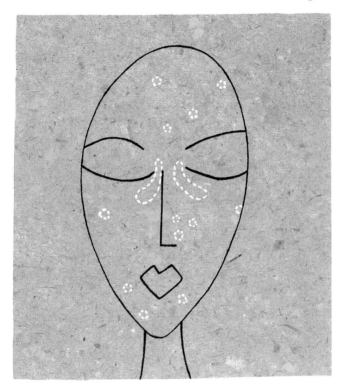

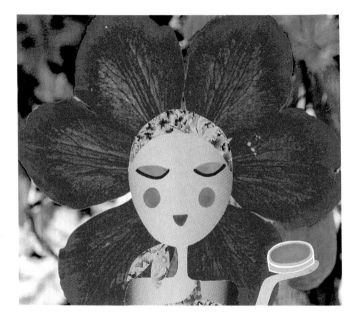

70 **Your best blusher color is the same shade as your natural skin tone after exerting yourself.** So run for a bus and then check your cheeks, or if you're feeling lazy, your natural lip color is also a good starting point. For a natural, healthy glow, always apply blusher to where you'd normally blush—the apples of your cheeks. Smile and brush on with an upward sweep, but don't get carried away. Blusher caught in your hairline is a dead giveaway. A touch on eyelids will also give you a quick healthy lift. Always make sure that blusher is the last item of makeup that you apply, so you can see exactly how much you need.

71 Use powder only on the parts of you that shine. And go for a yellow-toned product; translucent powder can drain color from your face.

72 Eyeliner pencil needs to be just the right temperature to do the job properly. Keep yours in the refrigerator during summer so it doesn't go too soft, and warm up the point on the back of your hand in winter if it gets too hard. For the best staying power, use a sponge-tipped applicator to apply a tiny bit of loose powder to your lid before using eyeliner. Or follow with an eye shadow in the same shade to set the color.

73 Too-dark brows will make your face look harder. Lighten them with a facial hair bleach (follow the manufacturer's instructions carefully) to instantly open up your eyes.

74 Eyebrow pencil can look too harsh when drawn directly on. Instead, rub the pencil on the back of your hand and then use a cotton swab to transfer it to your brows. And choose a shade that is slightly lighter than your own hair for a more natural look.

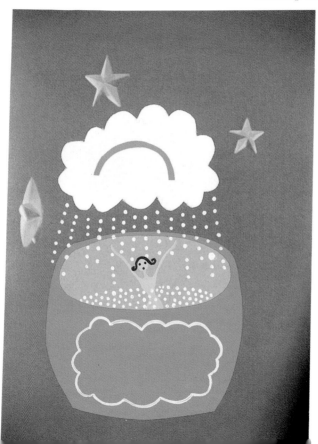

75 A small spray bottle of water is your makeup's best friend. A fine misting will instantly freshen up makeup that you've been wearing all day and will help set a newly applied face.

76 Some days your face just doesn't look like it should. For those nightmare mornings, rev up circulation with a scrub and then apply extra moisturizer to plump up your skin. Avoid foundation since this can make tired skin look even more exhausted and use concealer only where you need it (everywhere?) A pink blusher will do more than any other makeup to brighten your skin, and neutral eye shadow and lipstick will add warmth to your face. The biggest bad-day beauty mistake? Trying to overcompensate for your pale face by heaping on bright colors. You won't look any healthier, but you *will* look like a painted doll.

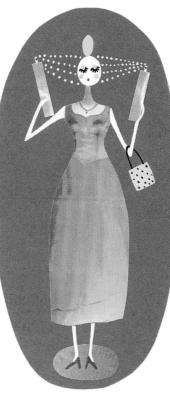

77 If you can't bear to go out bare-faced, choose waterproof products for swimming or active sports. Anything creamy will repel water, which means that a good, gooey lipstick, creamy or stick concealer, and cream blusher should be up to the job. If you are very active, consider dying your eyelashes to give you color without the risk of smearing (get this done professionally for the safest results). Or curl your lashes and brush on one coat of brown waterproof mascara. But be careful to keep your hands away from your eyes—these products are waterproof, but not smudgeproof.

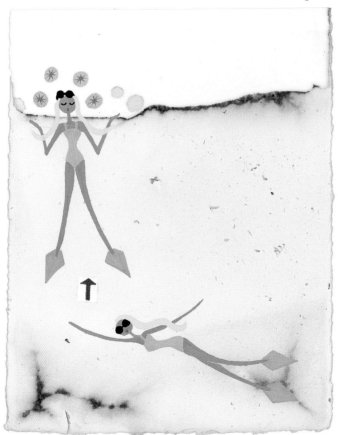

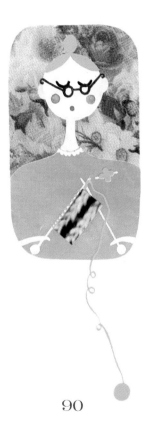

90

78 **As your face gets older, you need different makeup techniques to keep a youthful look.** For skin that's beginning to wrinkle, less is most definitely more. Apply a moisturizing foundation only where you need coverage and steer clear of lined areas or you'll just accentuate them. Go for cream eye shadows, cream blushers, and rich-moisture lipsticks (line your mouth first with a lip pencil to avoid feathering). And powder with caution: There's nothing more aging than powder settling into fine lines. Cake it on and you'll quickly turn a crease into a crevice.

79 **For the most natural look for older skin,** combine moisturizer with everything.

80 **Wake up tired-looking eyes with a dot of silver shadow** just on the inner corners of each eye. Or apply a little foundation to the same spot; it will also make your eyes look brighter.

91

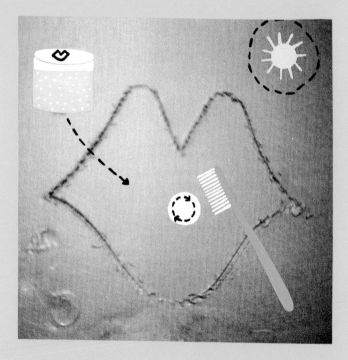

chapter 5

Perfect pout

81 **Nothing sets a pout off like set of perfect pearly white teeth**—keep yours in top condition by seeing your dentist every six months. That way your appointments will be for check-ups, not extractions!

82 **The four simple steps to healthy teeth:**

1. Use a toothpaste that contains fluoride, which helps protect your teeth from decay. When choosing dental products, look for the American Dental Association Seal of Acceptance.

2. Hold your brush at a 45 degree angle against your teeth and work backwards and forwards with short gentle strokes. Brush your gums gently at the same angle. Brush the inner and outer tooth surfaces, as well as the chewing surfaces of the teeth. Finally, brush your tongue to remove bacteria and freshen your breath.

3. Floss every time you brush, making sure you work away from the gums. Use a long piece of floss and feed it through your fingers so you're always using a clean part.

4. After brushing, rinse with a mouthwash to freshen breath and kill bacteria. Swish around your gums for about 30 seconds and then spit out.

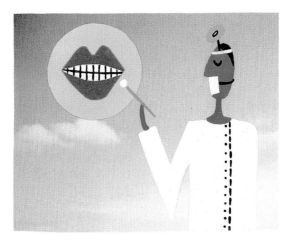

83 **Gum disease has taken over from tooth decay as the most frequent cause of tooth loss,** but fortunately this can largely be avoided by improving your cleaning habits. The average person spends less than 20 seconds brushing his or her teeth, which isn't long enough to stimulate the gums and remove plaque build-up. Increase your brushing time to a full two minutes and replace your toothbrush every two to three months; don't wait until the bristles wear out! Alternatively, invest in an electric toothbrush, which reaches between your teeth and below the gumline. Up to 90 percent of all plaque is removed in one scrub (more than twice as much as with an ordinary toothbrush).

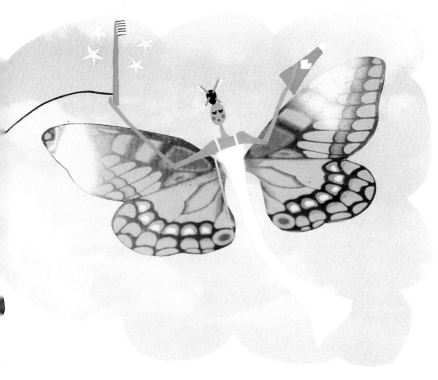

84 **Sugar is bad for your teeth as it reacts with plaque to form acids and toxins**—the main causes of gum disease and tooth decay. Cut down or cut out refined sugars in your diet, but also beware of natural sweeteners like glucose, dextrose, maltose, and fructose. Even more terrible for teeth are foods that stick fast, like chocolate and gooey caramel.

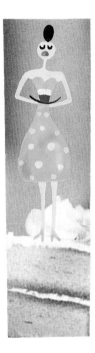

Chew on crunchy vegetables and fruit instead of snacking on candies and chocolate, and your teeth will thank you for it. Research has also shown that chewing unsweetened gum for 20 minutes after a meal, while no substitute for brushing, can stimulate saliva production to help fight plaque bacteria. Or instead of gum, try following the Asian tradition of chewing fennel and cardamom seeds after meals to prevent tooth decay, gum disease, and to sweeten breath.

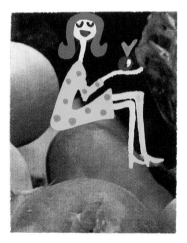

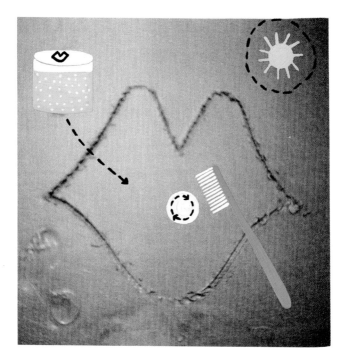

85 **Dry lips love a scrub. Slap on lots of petroleum jelly and then use an old toothbrush in small circular movements to lift off dry skin.** Or get under the shower and let lots of warm water run over your lips, then take a washcloth and gently rub over the surface. This has the double function of exfoliating dead skin while the water plumps up your pout. Finish off with a few dabs of lip balm.

86 **If your lips are dry and flaky, lightly wet them and then press on a piece of cellophane tape.** Gently peel off and all the cracked bits of skin will come away too.

87 **If you suffer from very dry lips, apply a nongreasy lip balm rather than a moisturizer—** which isn't designed for lips and will just make matters worse. To add color to dry lips, mix some of your favorite lipstick with a little lip balm using a lip brush, and gently dot onto your lips with your index finger for a fresh-faced look.

101

88 **The skin on your lips is thinner and lower in melanin (pigment) than on the rest of your face**, so it needs extra protection from sun, wind, and cold. To keep your lips looking luscious, protect them with a lip balm containing a sunscreen.

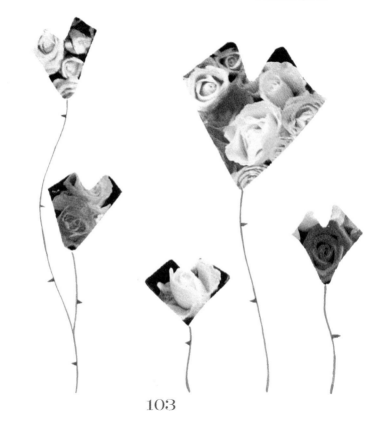

89 **Choose a lipstick to suit your skin and hair tones:**

Pale skin/dark hair: Create a contrast with fuchsia, red, or orange.

Fair skin/light hair: Go for browny beiges with complexion-warming pink or peach bases.

Dark skins: Be brave with dark blue-reds or deep wine-browns.

Olive skin/dark hair: Light-brown shades will light up your face.

Very pale or dark skins should avoid pale and pastel shades—they'll make you look like you're just getting over a bout of the flu!

90 **Nontransferable lipstick comes down to technique.** If your lips are dry, start by applying a little lip balm and let it absorb thoroughly. Next, build up the depth of shade by brushing on three thin coats of color, blotting with a tissue in between. For a final booster blot, separate a two-ply tissue, rest one half over your lips and dust on a little loose powder. To seal your lipstick and give extra shine, slick vitamin E oil over all.

91 **Banish bleeding lipstick by dabbing a little concealer onto a brush** and outlining your lips before you apply color. This will seal off any escape routes.

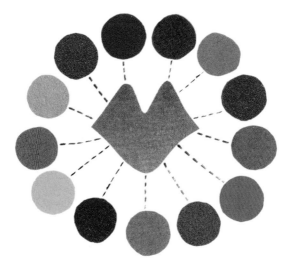

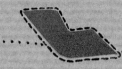

Pale colors make thin lips look thicker.

Dark colors make thin lips look thinner.

Pale colors make full lips look fatter.

Dark colors make full lips look more sophisticated.

Matte colors minimize lips.

Shiny colors magnify lips.

93 **Since the 1950s, red has been the choice of showbiz starlets.** Wearing red draws attention to your mouth, and it's said that men find it supersexy, since the color mimics the natural flush of passion. Don't shy away from red: The modern way to wear it is with very little other makeup or as a subtle stain— and there's a red for everyone:

• *Bright reds = all skin tones*
• *Orange reds = fair skin and blue eyes*
• *Mahogany reds = dark skin*
• *Blue reds = brunettes*
• *Brown reds = redheads*

94 **For a lip color straight out of the refrigerator,** wipe the cut side of a small piece of beet over your lips, or dab on a little red food coloring using a cotton swab. Much cheaper than any cosmetic.

95 **If you want your lips to look more luscious,** dab on a dot of lip gloss in the center of your bottom lip. As it catches the light, so will you!

96 **Outlining your lips with a skin-toned pencil before applying lipstick** will help to make them look larger. Taking the line just a little over your natural one will make your lips look larger still.

97 **Another makeup artist's trick for boosting the pout of thin-lipped models** is to apply a dab of concealer on the center of the bottom lip. This makes both lips look fuller as it brightens the lipstick one crucial shade, which catches the light.

98 **Lip liner sharpens the shape of your mouth and helps your lipstick stay on longer**, especially if you use it all over your lips. For a long-lasting natural look, finish with clear lip gloss.

99 **Fed up of finding lipstick on your teeth?** Copy a model trick and stick your index finger in your mouth, close your lips around it and pull your finger out. Any excess lipstick will stick to your skin on your finger not to your teeth.

100 **Oil-based makeup removers are best for wiping away waxy lipstick**, but other oils will have the same effect. Be warned—don't spend ages on your pout only to tuck into a plate of pesto pasta!

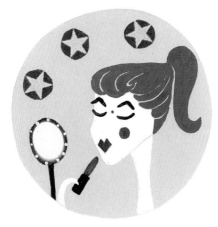

TIME® LIFE BOOKS

Time-Life Books is a division of Time Life Inc.

TIME LIFE INC.
Chairman and CEO   Jim Nelson
President and COO   Steven L. Janas

TIME-LIFE TRADE PUBLISHING
Vice President and Publisher   Neil Levin
Senior Director of Acquisitions
    and Editorial Resources   Jennifer Pearce
Director of New Product
    Development   Carolyn Clark
Director of Marketing   Inger Forland
Director of Trade Sales   Dana Hobson
Director of Custom Publishing   John Lalor
Director of Special Markets   Robert Lombardi
Director of Design   Kate L. McConnell
Project Manager   Jennifer L. Ward

TIME-LIFE is a trademark of Time Warner Inc. and
affiliated companies.

Books produced by Time-Life Trade Publishing are
available at a special bulk discount for promotional
and premium use. Custom adaptations can also be
created to meet your specific marketing goals.
Call 1-800-323-5255.

Cover design: Broadbase
Interior design: The Big Idea
Series editor: Elizabeth Carr

Printed in Hong Kong
10 9 8 7 6 5 4 3 2 1

Library of Congress Cataloging-in-Publication Data
Morley, Carol.
    Face : 100 makeup moves / Carol Morley,
Liz Wilde.
        p. cm.-- (Handbag honeys)
        ISBN 0-7370-0086-4 (hardcover)
    1. Beauty, Personal. 2. Face--Care and hygiene.
    3. Skin--Care and hygiene. 4. Cosmetics. I. Wilde,
Liz. II. Title. III. Series.

RA778 .M7695 2000
646.7'26--dc21   00-034354